Genuine Food for Fertility

Organic Nutrient-Rich Supplement

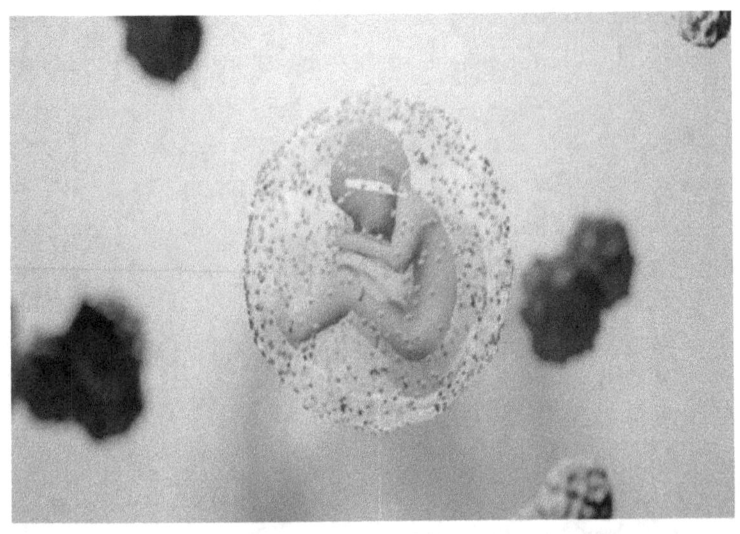

Mildred R. Thomas

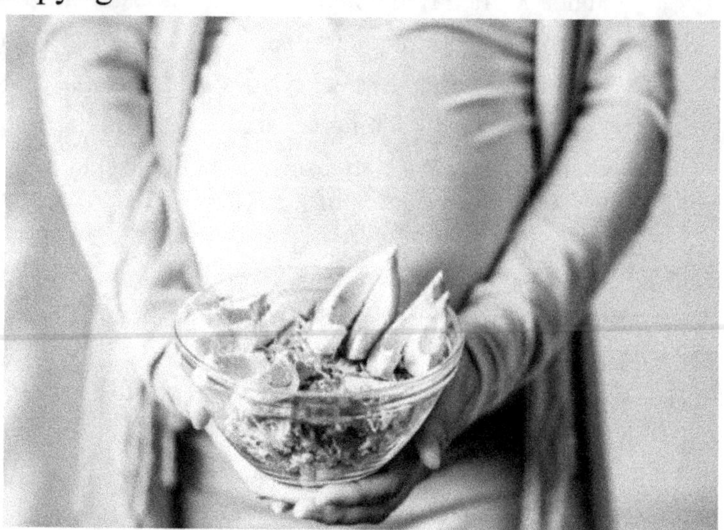

INTRODUCTION

Introduction to Genuine Food for Fertility

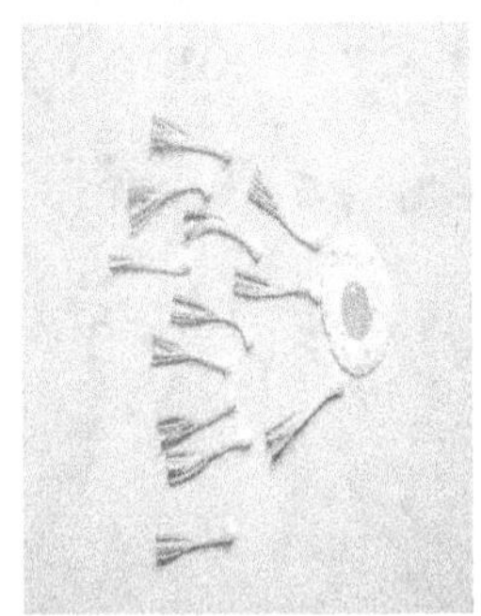

In the complicated fabric of human existence, the desire for a family frequently takes center stage, making fertility an extremely important issue. As couples start on the path to motherhood, they frequently investigate numerous options to improve their chances of pregnancy. One such option, which is sometimes underestimated, is the impact of authentic and nutritious cuisine in encouraging fertility.

Genuine food for fertility is more than just nutrition; it is the foundation for building a healthy environment within the body. The importance of diet in fertility is highlighted by the fact that the human body's complex reproductive system requires a careful balance of necessary nutrients, vitamins, and minerals to function optimally.

This road to fertility with authentic food takes a comprehensive approach to nutrition. It entails not just choosing nutrient-dense diets, but also comprehending the substantial influence these decisions can have on reproductive health. Genuine foods, in this perspective, are entire, unprocessed, and minimally refined choices that preserve their original deliciousness.

Researchers and healthcare professionals have been more interested in the relationship between food and fertility. According to research, some nutrients serve critical roles in sustaining reproductive health, controlling hormonal balance, and establishing a favourable environment for conception. Antioxidants, omega-3 fatty acids, vitamins, and minerals all play a role in the body's complex fertility dance.

As we go into the area of real food for fertility, this exploration intends to shed light on the foods that can help improve reproductive health. From colorful fruits and vegetables to lean proteins, nutritious grains, and fertility-friendly fats, the route to pregnancy becomes inextricably linked to the food choices we make every day.

Starting down the path of true food for fertility is more than merely checking off a list of necessary nutrients. It is a commitment to nurture both the body and the mind, providing the framework for a successful reproductive journey. Through this investigation, we hope to give insights, assistance, and a better understanding of the significant connection between authentic dietary choices and the delicate tapestry of fertility.

Preconception

Preconception diet is critical for laying the groundwork for a successful pregnancy and improving the health of both the mother and the future baby. Planning a pregnancy is more than just stopping contraception; it also entails paying attention to dietary choices, which can have a substantial influence on fertility, fetal development, and long-term health results. Here are some important factors to consider when it comes to preconception nutrition:

Folic Acid:

Adequate folic acid consumption prior to conception and throughout the first weeks of pregnancy can lower the incidence of neural tube abnormalities in the developing baby. Fortified cereals, leafy green vegetables, legumes, and healthcare professional-recommended supplements are all good sources of folic acid.

Healthy weight:

Maintaining a healthy weight before to conception is vital for both spouses. Being underweight or overweight might impair fertility and increase the likelihood of pregnancy problems.

A balanced diet and regular physical activity help you achieve and maintain a healthy weight.

Balanced Diet:

A well-balanced diet that includes fruits, vegetables, whole grains, lean meats, and dairy products provides a wide range of vital elements.

Iron, calcium, vitamin D, and omega-3 fatty acids are essential for reproductive health and embryonic development.

Limiting your exposure to harmful substances:

Tobacco, alcohol, recreational drugs, and some environmental pollutants should be avoided or minimized in order to maintain good preconception health.

Both couples should work to avoid or limit their exposure to these drugs in order to promote fertility and lower the chance of birth abnormalities.

Caffeine and Alcohol Intake:

Moderation is essential when it comes to coffee and alcohol usage. Caffeine has been linked to reproductive problems, whilst heavy alcohol use might raise the chance of miscarriage and birth abnormalities.
Both spouses should minimize their caffeine and alcohol intake before and throughout pregnancy.

Supplementation:

In addition to folic acid, healthcare experts may offer iron, calcium, and vitamin D supplements based on individual requirements.

Prenatal vitamins can help ensure that the mother gets enough nutrients, especially in the early stages of pregnancy when nutritional requirements increase.

Regular Exercise:

Regular physical activity improves overall health and helps you maintain a healthy weight. It can also reduce stress, increase mood, and promote conception.

However, excessive exercise can have a detrimental impact on fertility, so striking a balance is essential.

Before attempting to conceive, both spouses should have preconception check-ups with their doctors. These visits can address underlying health concerns, evaluate nutritional status, and make individualized suggestions.

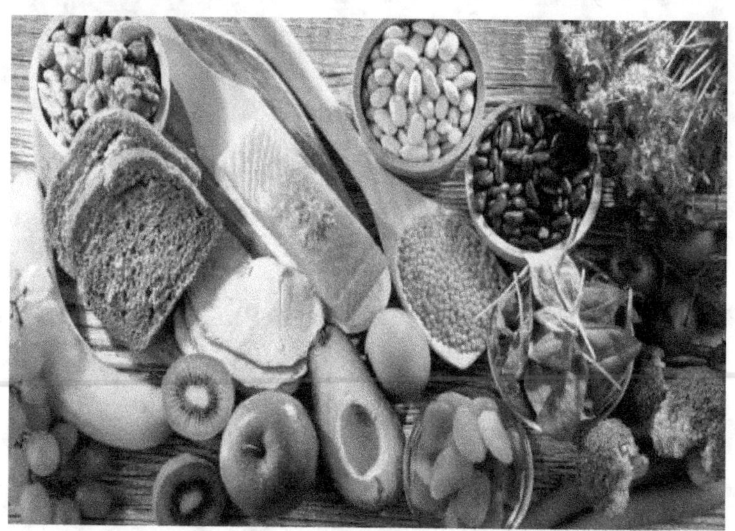

CHAPTER 1: INTRODUCTION TO FERTILITY AND FOOD

Unveiling the Power of Food for Optimal Fertility

Fertility is a complicated and delicate component of human health that is affected by a variety of factors including lifestyle, genetics, and diet. While medical therapies are essential, the influence of nutrition on fertility should not be overlooked. This article looks at the important impact that food can have in fostering good fertility.

Nutrient-Rich Diet:

A well-balanced, nutrient-rich diet promotes general health and fertility. Include a mix of fruits and vegetables, whole grains, lean proteins, and healthy fats in your daily diet. These foods include vital vitamins, minerals, and antioxidants that promote reproductive health.

Folate and Fertility:

Folate, a B-vitamin, is essential for fertility, particularly for women trying to conceive. It has been shown to lessen the likelihood of neural tube abnormalities in babies. Leafy greens, citrus fruits, and legumes are rich in folate and should be included in a fertility-focused diet.

Omega-3 Fatty Acids:

Omega-3 fatty acids promote reproductive health. These fatty acids, found in fatty fish, flaxseeds, and walnuts, help to regulate hormone synthesis and reduce inflammation, resulting in a healthy reproductive system.

Adequate Protein Intake:

Protein is essential for cellular, tissue, and hormone function. Consume a proper amount of lean protein sources such as poultry, fish, beans, and tofu. Protein contributes to the formation of healthy eggs and sperm.

Choose complex carbs, such whole grains, over processed carbohydrates. These carbs have a lower glycemic index, which aids in blood sugar regulation and insulin resistance, both of which have been associated with fertility concerns.

Maintaining proper hydration is crucial for optimal health and fertility. Water serves to carry nutrients, control body temperature, and provide a healthy environment for reproductive cells.

Limit Processed Foods and Sugar:

Limit processed foods and sugar intake, as they can cause inflammation and hormone imbalances. Reduce your usage of processed foods, sugary beverages, and refined sugars to promote healthy fertility.

Maintain a Healthy Weight:

Both being underweight and overweight might negatively impact fertility. Strive to maintain a healthy weight by combining a good diet with frequent exercise. Consult a healthcare expert for specific guidance.

Antioxidant-Rich Foods:

Antioxidants protect reproductive cells from free radicals. To maintain the health of eggs and sperm, eat antioxidant-rich foods like berries, almonds, and colorful vegetables.

Understanding Your Fertility: The Cycle, Your Body, and You

Fertility is a complex and fascinating feature of human biology, with a critical role in the life cycle. Individuals and couples who want to conceive should get a better grasp of the complex processes that occur within the female reproductive system. In this examination, we'll look at the menstrual cycle, the many stages of fertility, and how your body signals its preparation for conception.

The Cycle

The fertility cycle is a dynamic and sophisticated process that occurs within the female reproductive system, coordinating the possibility for pregnancy. This cyclical trip is largely governed by hormones and occurs in several stages, with each playing an important part in the overall fertility landscape.

Menstruation (days 1–5):

Menstruation, or the shedding of the uterine lining if fertilization did not occur in the previous cycle, begins the cycle.

Hormone levels are at their lowest, causing the body to prepare for the formation of a new egg.

Follicular Phase (Days 6–14):

The pituitary gland secretes follicle-stimulating hormone (FSH), which stimulates the ovaries to create multiple follicles.

One dominant follicle develops and grows, producing estrogen and thickening the uterine lining.

Ovulation (day 14):

Ovulation is the apex of fertility, occurring around the 14th day of a typical 28-day cycle. Luteinizing hormone (LH) levels rise, signaling the release of the mature egg from the ovary, making it ready for fertilization.

Luteal Phase (Days 15 to 28):

The burst follicle develops into the corpus luteum, which is a transitory endocrine tissue that generates progesterone.

Progesterone prepares the uterine lining for a prospective embryo and creates a favorable environment for early pregnancy.

Implantation or menstruation:

If fertilization takes place, the fertilized egg travels down the fallopian tube and implants in the uterus.

If fertilization does not occur, hormone levels fall, resulting in the loss of the uterine lining and the start of a new cycle.

Understanding fertility entails identifying the signals and processes in your body that suggest the possibility of pregnancy. Here are crucial factors to consider:

Menstrual Cycle:

Track your menstrual cycle to determine its duration and regularity. The menstrual cycle lasts around 28 days, however it varies from woman to woman.

Ovulation, or the release of an egg from the ovary, often happens in the middle of the menstrual cycle. This is frequently regarded as the most fruitful season.

Base Body Temperature (BBT):

Record your basal body temperature by taking it every morning before getting out of bed. A modest rise in temperature (0.5-1°F) following ovulation shows that ovulation has occurred.

Cervical mucus:

Pay attention to cervical mucous changes. Around ovulation, cervical mucus becomes transparent, slick, and elastic, similar to the nature of egg whites. This promotes sperm mobility.

Ovulation predictor kits (OPKs):

Use ovulation predictor kits to identify the spike in luteinizing hormone (LH) that occurs before ovulation. These kits can help you determine which days of your cycle are the most fertile.

Menstrual pain:

During ovulation, some women suffer mittelschmerz, which is minor pelvic discomfort or cramping. This might be another sign of fertility.

Libido and Sensation:

Increased libido or heightened feelings may occur around ovulation, potentially due to hormonal changes.

Regular health checkups:

Regular health examinations are recommended to address any underlying fertility difficulties, such as hormone imbalances or reproductive abnormalities.

Age and Lifestyle Factors:

Understand that age influences fertility, with peak fertility happening in the early to mid-20s and steadily dropping after that.
Diet, exercise, stress, and drug use are among lifestyle variables that might affect fertility.

Consult with a Healthcare Professional:

If you're actively trying to conceive and have difficulties, speak with a healthcare provider or a fertility expert. They can give individualized guidance, testing, and fertility treatments if necessary.

Building the Foundation: Creating a Healthy Lifestyle for Fertility

Developing a healthy lifestyle is critical for increasing fertility. Here are a few techniques to promote fertility through lifestyle choices:

Balanced Diet:

Eat a well-balanced diet high in fruits and vegetables, whole grains, lean meats, and healthy fats.

Maintain an appropriate diet of important nutrients such as folic acid, iron, zinc, and vitamins.

Maintain a healthy weight:

Aim for a healthy body weight, since both obesity and underweight can impair fertility. Regular exercise can help you reach and maintain a healthy weight.

Regular Exercise:

Engage in moderate, frequent activity, such as brisk walking or swimming, to improve general health and fertility.
Avoid excessive or strenuous activity, as this might interrupt the menstrual cycle.

Manage stress:

Practice stress-relieving practices such as yoga, meditation, deep breathing, and mindfulness.

Chronic stress can disrupt reproductive hormones and menstrual cycles.

Adequate Sleep:

Ensure enough and high-quality sleep (7-9 hours each night) to maintain hormonal balance and promote general well-being.

Limit alcohol and caffeine:

Consume alcohol in moderation and restrict caffeine usage, as large quantities might impair fertility.

Quit smoking:

Quit smoking, since it reduces fertility in both men and women and raises the risk of miscarriage.

Stay hydrated:

Drink enough water to keep hydrated, which promotes general health and reproductive function.

Regular Health Check-Ups:

Schedule frequent check-ups with your healthcare practitioner to analyze and screen your reproductive health.

Avoid environmental toxins:

Reduce your exposure to environmental pollutants, such as pesticides and chemicals, which can affect fertility.

Fertility-friendly lubricants:

Use fertility-friendly lubricants as necessary, as some can impair sperm motility.

Understand the Menstrual Cycle:

Track and understand your menstrual cycle to determine peak fertility days for conception.

Limit processed foods:

Reduce your consumption of processed meals, sugary snacks, and beverages, since they may lead to inflammation and hormone abnormalities.

Include omega-3 fatty acids:

To promote reproductive health, eat omega-3 fatty acid-rich foods like fish, flaxseeds, and walnuts.

Optimize vitamin D levels:

Vitamin D is important for reproductive health and should be obtained from sunshine exposure and/or supplementation.

Practice safe sex:

Protect yourself from sexually transmitted infections (STIs) by engaging in safe sex, as certain illnesses might affect fertility.

Balanced hormones:

Maintain hormonal balance via a healthy lifestyle, as imbalances can impair ovulation and sperm production.

Consider prenatal supplements:

If you intend to conceive, begin taking prenatal vitamins containing folic acid and other vital nutrients before conception.

Moderate Caffeine Intake:

Caffeine usage should be moderate, as high consumption has been linked to reproductive problems.

Mindful eating:

Practice mindful eating, paying attention to hunger and fullness cues while avoiding emotional or stress-related eating.

Stay informed:

Stay knowledgeable about your reproductive health, and be proactive in finding information about fertility and conception.

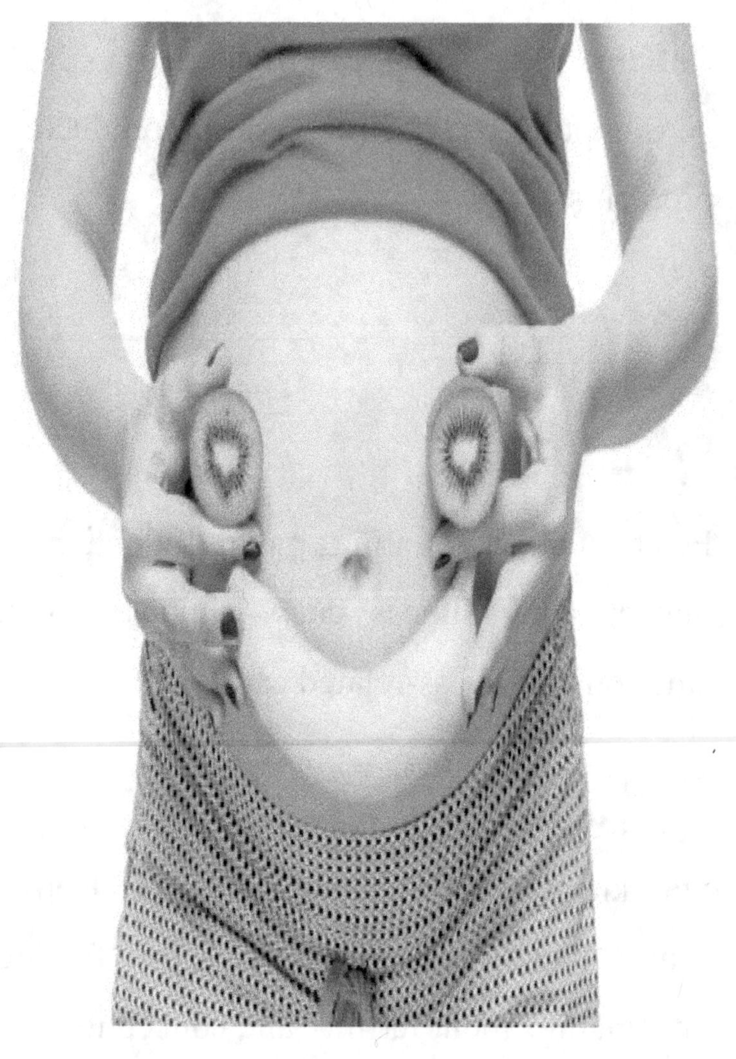

CHAPTER 2: NOURISHING YOUR BODY FOR CONCEPTION

The Fertility Plate: A Guide to Nutrient-Rich Eating.

Nutrition plays an important part in the process of conceiving and maintaining a healthy pregnancy. The Fertility Plate is a thorough guide to nutrient-rich nutrition, giving critical insights into boosting fertility with a well-balanced and healthy diet. By including critical nutrients into your meals, you may create an atmosphere that promotes reproductive health and well-being.

The Foundation of Fertility Nutrition

Understanding Nutritional Needs:

To begin on the path of fertility-focused nutrition, it is critical to understand the individual nutrients that play an important role in reproductive health. This section discusses the significance of macronutrients like protein, fat, and carbs, as well as micronutrients like vitamins and minerals.

The Effect of Lifestyle Factors:

Examine how lifestyle choices such as physical exercise, stress management, and appropriate sleep affect overall fertility. Learn how minor changes to everyday routines can have a significant influence on reproductive results.

Building the Fertility Plate

Powerhouse Fertility Foods:

Learn about nutrient-dense foods that can help with fertility, such as leafy greens, berries, nuts, seeds, and lean meats. This section provides practical strategies for incorporating these items into your everyday meals.

Balancing Macronutrients:

Optimal protein, fat, and carbohydrate balance for fertility requires high-quality sources and a balanced diet.

Key Nutrients for Reproductive Health.

Folate and Fertility:

Understand the importance of folate in preconception nutrition, including dietary sources and supplemental alternatives to promote fetal development and avoid neural tube abnormalities.

Omega-3 Fatty Acids:

 Learn how omega-3 fatty acids can improve fertility and pregnancy outcomes. Consider foods like fatty salmon, flaxseeds, and walnuts.

Understand the role of iron in avoiding anemia during pregnancy and discover iron-rich foods for a fertility-focused diet.

Meal Plans and Recipes

Creating Fertility-Friendly Recipes:

Receive practical advice on meal planning to maximize fertility, including example meal plans and tasty food options that adhere to fertility nutrition principles.

Supercharging Your Eggs: Essential Nutrients for Optimal Health.

Achieving optimal reproductive health requires a variety of lifestyle decisions, including eating. Women who want to conceive must ensure the health and viability of their ova (eggs). Supercharging your ovum entails putting vital nutrients into your diet to promote overall reproductive health. In this article, we'll look at crucial nutrients that can help improve the health of your eggs and increase fertility.

Folate and folic acid.

Folate, a B-vitamin, is required for DNA synthesis and repair, ensuring the formation of healthy eggs. Folic acid, a synthetic version of folate, is frequently advised for women trying to conceive. Leafy greens, citrus fruits, and fortified cereals are all good providers of these nutrients.

Omega 3 Fatty Acids:

Omega-3 fatty acids, particularly DHA and EPA, are critical to reproductive health. They maintain hormonal balance and promote healthy cellular activity. To increase your omega-3 levels, eat more fatty fish, flaxseeds, chia seeds, and walnuts.

Antioxidants:

Oxidative stress can reduce egg quality. Antioxidants include vitamins C and E, selenium, and beta-carotene aid to neutralize free radicals. Colorful fruits and vegetables, nuts, seeds, and whole grains are high in antioxidants.

Iron:

Adequate iron levels are necessary for proper blood flow to the reproductive organs. Red meat, chicken, beans, and fortified cereals can help the body maintain proper iron levels.

Vitamin D:

Vitamin D is necessary for hormonal balance and good reproductive health. Sun exposure, fatty fish, and fortified dairy products are all good sources of vitamin D.

Protein:

Protein is a fundamental building ingredient for all organisms, including eggs. To promote healthy ova development, consume lean protein sources such as poultry, fish, tofu, and lentils.

Iodine:

Iodine is essential for thyroid function, which helps regulate reproductive hormones. Iodine-rich foods include seafood, dairy products, and iodized salt.

Zinc:

Zinc is involved in DNA synthesis and cell division, hence it is essential for the creation of viable eggs. Consume zinc-rich foods such as lean meats, dairy products, and nuts.

Calcium:

Calcium is necessary for general bone health and can help to keep reproductive organs functioning properly. Calcium-rich foods include leafy greens, dairy products, and fortified plant-based milk.

Hydration:

Staying hydrated is critical for general health, including reproductive health. Adequate water consumption promotes nutrition delivery and helps to maintain normal physiological processes.

Empowering Sperm: Foods to Enhance
Quality and Motility

In the quest of reproductive health, both men and women play important responsibilities. For males, the quality and motility of sperm are critical variables in fertility. Lifestyle decisions, especially food, can have a substantial influence on sperm health. This book investigates the empowering properties of specific meals that have been shown to improve sperm quality and motility.

Fatty Fish: Omega-3 Rich Delights:
Fatty fish, like salmon, mackerel, and sardines, are high in omega-3 fatty acids.

These critical lipids are necessary for sperm development and function. Omega-3s help to maintain the structural integrity of sperm cells and improve overall reproductive health. Including fish in your diet might be a tasty and healthy method to improve sperm count.

Colorful fruits and vegetables : Antioxidant Powerhouses.

A diet high in fruits and vegetables contains several antioxidants that battle oxidative stress. Oxidative stress can harm sperm DNA and impair motility. Berries, citrus fruits, tomatoes, and leafy greens are high in vitamins and antioxidants, which defend against free radicals and promote healthy sperm function.

Nuts and Seeds: A Protein and Nutrient-Rich Snack

Nuts and seeds, including walnuts, almonds, and sunflower seeds, are high in vital elements including zinc, selenium, and vitamin E. These nutrients play critical functions in sperm health. Zinc, in particular, is known to improve sperm motility and preserve the integrity of the sperm cell membrane.

Whole Grains: Fuel for Sperm Production.

Whole grains, such as oats, brown rice, and quinoa, are high in complex carbs and give a steady supply of energy. This energy is essential for the ongoing process of sperm generation. Furthermore, whole grains include selenium, which promotes healthy sperm growth and motility.

Leafy greens include folate, which promotes DNA integrity.

Leafy greens, like spinach and kale, are high in folate, a B-vitamin required for DNA synthesis and repair. Maintaining DNA integrity is critical for proper sperm growth. Including folate-rich foods in your diet can help to reduce genetic abnormalities in sperm and promote overall reproductive success.

Lean Proteins: Building Blocks of Sperm

Lean protein foods, such as poultry, lean beef, and tofu, include amino acids required for sperm synthesis. Protein is an important building ingredient for the formation of sperm cells. A well-balanced diet rich in lean protein provides the body with the nutrients it requires for optimum sperm production.

Balancing Blood Sugar: The Key to Hormonal Harmony

In the delicate dance of our bodies' internal systems, hormone balance is critical to sustaining general health and well-being. Blood sugar management is an often neglected but critical component of this delicate balance. The interaction between blood sugar levels and hormonal balance is a complicated but necessary relationship that affects a variety of body activities. Understanding how to manage blood sugar is critical for maintaining hormonal homeostasis and supporting general health.

The Blood Sugar and Hormone Connection:

The pancreas produces insulin and glucagon, which play a crucial role in regulating blood sugar levels. Insulin promotes glucose absorption into cells, which lowers blood sugar levels, whereas glucagon raises blood sugar levels by releasing stored glucose when necessary. The dynamic interaction of these hormones is critical for maintaining stable blood sugar levels.

Chronic blood sugar abnormalities can alter the regulation of cortisol, the stress hormone. Elevated cortisol levels, which are commonly caused by unstable blood sugar, can lead to weight gain, insulin resistance, and irregular menstrual cycles in women. Balancing blood sugar helps to attenuate these effects and promotes overall hormonal balance.

Thyroid Function: The thyroid gland regulates hormones and is sensitive to blood sugar levels. Fluctuations in blood sugar can impair thyroid function, potentially leading to hypothyroidism or hyperthyroidism. Stable blood sugar levels promote good thyroid function and hormonal balance.

Strategies for Managing Blood Sugar:

A nutrient-dense diet: with whole foods, lean proteins, and complex carbs can help regulate blood sugar levels. Avoiding refined sugars and processed meals is critical for preventing rapid blood sugar spikes and falls.

Regular physical: activity promotes glucose metabolism and insulin sensitivity. Both aerobic and resistance exercise help to maintain stable blood sugar levels and promote hormonal balance.

 Prolonged stress might increase cortisol levels, affecting blood sugar control. Stress-reduction techniques such as meditation, deep breathing, and proper sleep can help improve hormonal balance.

 throughout the day can help manage blood sugar levels. Avoiding extended fasting or overeating can help maintain stable glucose levels and hormonal balance.

 promotes general health and helps maintain stable blood sugar levels. Water facilitates nutrition transfer and promotes the body's natural activities, such as hormone control.

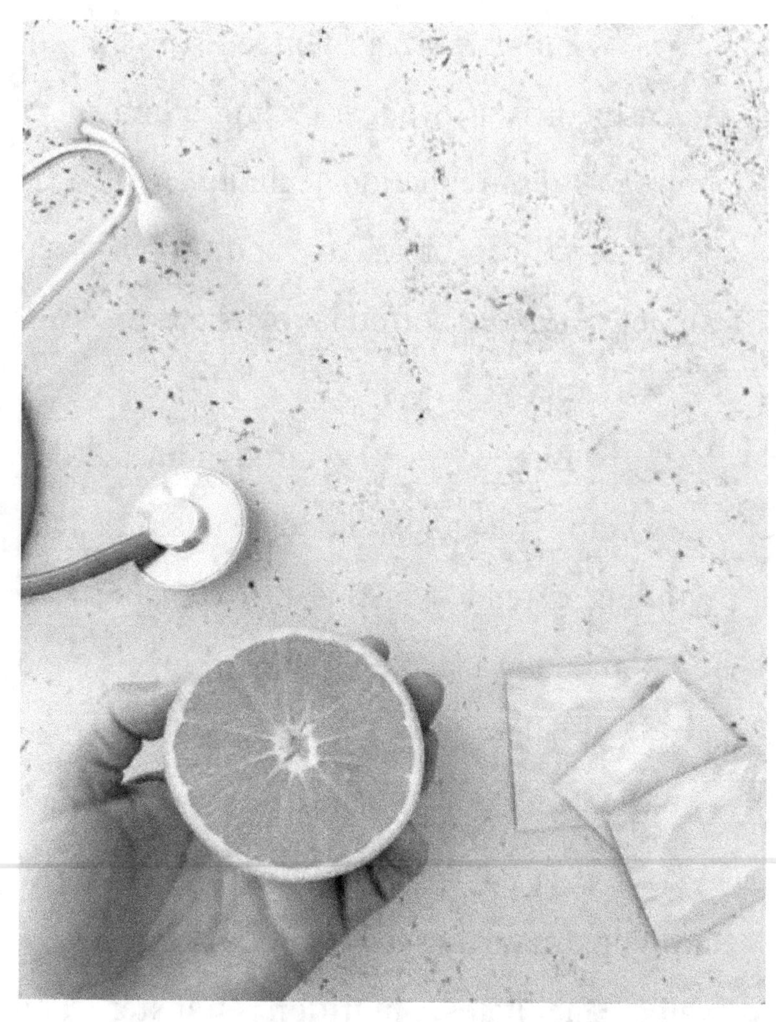

CHAPTER 3: PUTTING YOUR KNOWLEDGE INTO PRACTICE

Sample Meal Plans for Fertility Support

When preparing meals to enhance fertility, it is important to focus on a balanced and healthy diet.

Meal Plan 1: Balanced Diet

Breakfast:

- Quinoa Breakfast Bowl
- Cooked quinoa with mixed berries
- Greek yogurt
- Chia seeds
- Walnuts or almonds

Lunch:

- Grilled Chicken Salad
- Mixed greens (spinach, kale, arugula)
- Grilled chicken breast
- Avocado slices
- Cherry tomatoes
- Olive oil and lemon dressing

Snack:

- Greek Yogurt Parfait
- Greek yogurt
- Honey
- Granola
- Mixed fruits (berries, kiwi)

Dinner:

- Baked Salmon

- Wild-caught salmon fillet
- Quinoa or brown rice
- Steamed broccoli
- Lemon and dill sauce

Snack:

- Mixed Nuts
- Almonds, walnuts, pistachios
- Dried apricots or figs

Meal Plan 2: Plant-Based Option

Breakfast:

- Smoothie Bowl
- Spinach, banana, and berry smoothie
- Topped with sliced almonds and chia seeds

Lunch:

- Chickpea and Vegetable Stir-Fry
- Chickpeas
- Colorful bell peppers
- Broccoli
- Quinoa or brown rice
- Soy sauce and ginger dressing

Snack:

- Hummus with Veggie Sticks
- Carrot, cucumber, and bell pepper sticks
- Hummus for dipping

Dinner:

- Lentil and Sweet Potato Curry

- Red lentils

- Sweet potatoes

- Coconut milk

- Spices (turmeric, cumin, coriander)

- Quinoa or whole grain bread on the side

Snack:

- Fruit Salad

- Mixed fruits (pineapple, mango, berries)

Meal Plan 3: Mediterranean Inspired

Breakfast:

- Mediterranean Omelette
- Eggs with tomatoes, spinach, and feta cheese
- Whole grain toast
- Olive oil drizzle

Lunch:

- Quinoa Greek Salad
- Quinoa
- Cherry tomatoes
- Cucumber
- Kalamata olives
- Feta cheese
- Olive oil and lemon dressing

- Roasted Red Pepper Hummus with Whole Wheat Pita
- Sliced cucumber and carrot sticks

Dinner:

- Grilled Shrimp with Lemon and Garlic
- Brown rice or couscous
- Grilled asparagus
- Lemon wedges

Snack:

- Greek Yogurt with Honey and Berries

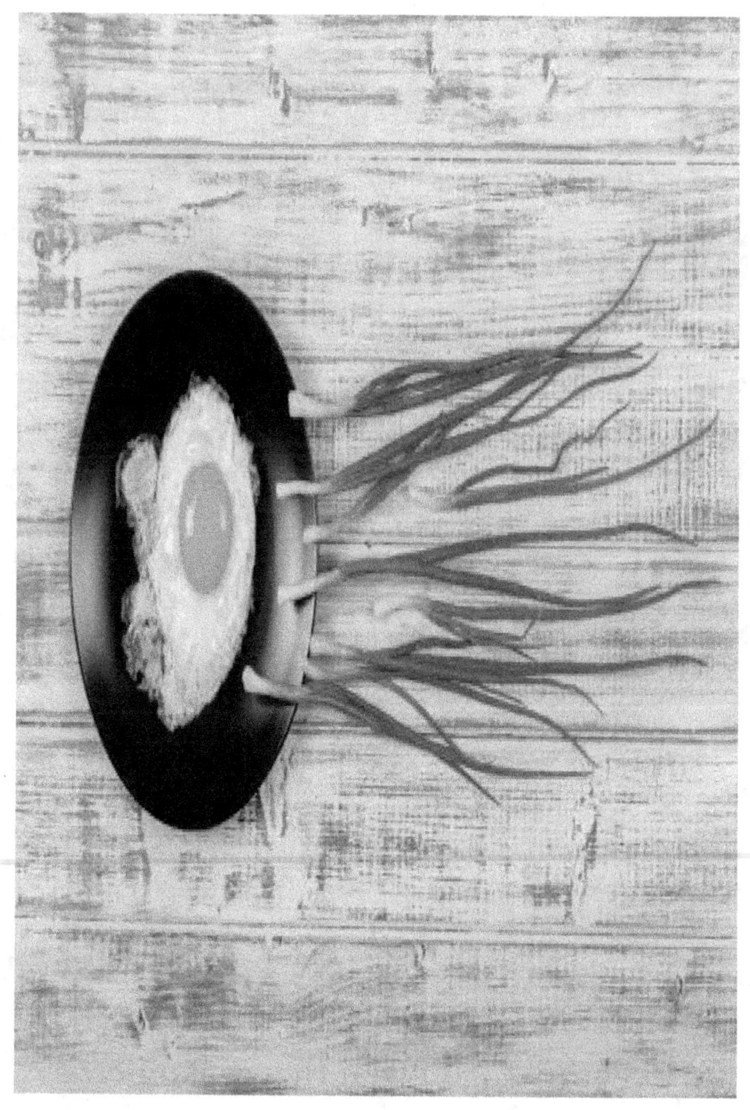

Meal Plan 4: High Protein Focus

Breakfast:

- Protein-Packed Smoothie
- Greek yogurt
- Banana
- Spinach
- Protein powder
- Almond milk

Lunch:

- Turkey and Avocado Wrap
- Whole grain wrap
- Sliced turkey breast
- Avocado
- Lettuce and tomato
- Greek yogurt-based dressing

Snack:

- Cottage Cheese with Pineapple
- Sprinkle with chia seeds

Dinner:

- Baked Chicken Breast
- Quinoa or sweet potato
- Steamed green beans
- Lemon and herb marinade

Snack:

- Hard-Boiled Eggs with a Sprinkle of Paprika

Meal Plan 5: Balanced Vegetarian Option

Breakfast:

- Overnight Chia Seed Pudding
- Chia seeds soaked in almond milk
- Mixed with sliced strawberries and a touch of honey
- Topped with chopped nuts

Lunch:

- Lentil and Vegetable Stuffed Bell Peppers
- Bell peppers stuffed with a mix of lentils, quinoa, tomatoes, and spices
- Side of mixed greens with balsamic vinaigrette

Snack:

- Apple Slices with Almond Butter

Dinner:

- Roasted Vegetable and Chickpea Buddha Bowl
- Roasted sweet potatoes, broccoli, and chickpeas
- Quinoa
- Tahini dressing

Snack:

- Mixed Berries with Cottage Cheese

Meal Plan 6: Omega-3 Rich Choices

Breakfast:

- Smoked Salmon and Avocado Toast

- Whole grain toast

- Smoked salmon

- Sliced avocado

- Lemon juice and dill

Lunch:

- Spinach and Walnut Salad

- Baby spinach leaves

- Grilled chicken or tofu

- Cherry tomatoes

- Feta cheese

- Toasted walnuts

- Balsamic vinaigrette

Snack:

- Flaxseed and Berry Smoothie

- Flaxseeds, mixed berries, Greek yogurt, and a splash of almond milk

Dinner:

- Baked Cod with Quinoa
- Cod filet seasoned with herbs
- Quinoa
- Steamed broccoli
- Olive oil and lemon drizzle

Snack:

- Greek Yogurt with Flaxseed and Honey.

Cooking for Fertility: Delicious and Nutritious Recipes

Starting a fertility journey frequently requires a comprehensive strategy, and diet is critical in supporting reproductive health. By including fertility-friendly products into your meals, you may provide a tasty and healthy foundation for your reproductive objectives. Here, we share a variety of recipes meant to improve fertility using the power of nutritious, nutrient-dense foods.

Fertility-Boosting Smoothie:

Ingredients:

- 1 cup mixed berries (blueberries, strawberries, raspberries)

- 1 ripe banana

- 1/2 cup Greek yogurt

- 1 tablespoon flaxseeds

- 1 tablespoon honey

- 1 cup spinach leaves

- 1/2 cup almond milk

Instructions:

- Blend all of the ingredients until smooth, then enjoy this nutrient-dense smoothie rich with antioxidants, omega-3 fatty acids, and vitamins.

Salmon and Quinoa Bowl:

Ingredients:

- 1 cup cooked quinoa

- 6 oz wild-caught salmon fillet
- 1 cup broccoli florets
- 1 tablespoon olive oil
- 1 clove garlic, minced
- Lemon juice, salt, and pepper to taste

Instructions:

- Season the salmon with olive oil, chopped garlic, salt, and pepper.
- Bake or grill the fish until done.
- Steam broccoli till tender.
- Fill the bowl with salmon, quinoa, and broccoli.
- Drizzle with lemon juice for extra taste.

Mango Avocado Salad:

Ingredients:

- 1 ripe mango, diced
- 1 ripe avocado, sliced
- 2 cups mixed greens
- 1/4 cup pumpkin seeds
- Feta cheese (optional)
- Balsamic vinaigrette dressing

Instructions:

- Mix mango, avocado, mixed greens, and pumpkin seeds in a dish.
- If desired, mix with crumbled feta cheese.
- To make a refreshing and nutrient-rich salad, drizzle with balsamic vinaigrette and gently mix.

Sweet Potato and Chickpea Curry:

Ingredients:

- 2 medium sweet potatoes, peeled and diced
- 1 can chickpeas, drained and rinsed
- 1 onion, chopped
- 2 cloves garlic, minced
- 1 can coconut milk
- 2 tablespoons curry powder
- Fresh cilantro for garnish

Instructions:

- Sauté the onion and garlic until tender.
- Combine sweet potatoes, chickpeas, coconut milk, and curry powder.

Simmer until the sweet potatoes are soft.

- Garnish with fresh cilantro before serving. This curry contains a good combination of protein, healthy fats, and complex carbs.

Ingredients:

- 1 cup mixed berries (strawberries, blueberries, raspberries)
- 1 cup Greek yogurt
- 1/4 cup granola
- Drizzle of honey

- In a glass or dish, combine Greek yogurt, mixed berries, and granola.
- Drizzle with honey for sweetness, and enjoy this fertility-boosting parfait high in probiotics, antioxidants, and vitamins.

Spinach and Mushroom Omelette:

Ingredients:

- 3 eggs
- 1 cup fresh spinach, chopped
- 1/2 cup mushrooms, sliced
- 1 tablespoon olive oil
- Salt and pepper to taste

- Sauté the mushrooms and spinach in olive oil until wilted.
- Whisk the eggs, then pour them over the veggies. Cook until set.
- This protein-packed omelette is high in folate and iron, which are essential for reproductive health.

Quinoa-Stuffed Bell Peppers:

Ingredients:

- 4 bell peppers, halved
- 1 cup cooked quinoa
- 1 can black beans, drained and rinsed
- 1 cup corn kernels
- 1 cup diced tomatoes

- 1 teaspoon cumin

- Shredded cheese (optional)

Instructions:

- Combine the quinoa, black beans, corn, tomatoes, and cumin in a bowl.

- Stuff bell peppers with the mixture and bake until they are soft.

- For a fertility-friendly, plant-based cuisine, sprinkle with shredded cheese if desired.

Lemon Garlic Shrimp Pasta:

Ingredients:

- 8 oz whole-grain pasta

- 1 lb shrimp, peeled and deveined
- 3 cloves garlic, minced
- Zest and juice of 1 lemon
- 2 tablespoons olive oil
- Fresh parsley for garnish

Instructions:

- Cook the pasta according to the package instructions.
- Sauté the shrimp and garlic in olive oil until they're done.
- Combine cooked pasta, shrimp, lemon zest, and lemon juice. Garnish with fresh parsley.

Cinnamon Roasted Sweet Potatoes:

Ingredients:

- 2 large sweet potatoes, peeled and cubed
- 2 tablespoons coconut oil, melted
- 1 teaspoon cinnamon
- 1/4 teaspoon nutmeg
- Pinch of salt

Instructions:

- Preheat the oven to 400 °F (200 °C).
- Combine sweet potatoes, melted coconut oil, cinnamon, nutmeg, and salt.
- Roast until tender, stirring periodically. These sweet potatoes include beta-carotene and fiber.

Berry Chia Seed Pudding:

Ingredients:

- 1/4 cup chia seeds
- 1 cup almond milk
- 1 teaspoon vanilla extract
- Mixed berries for topping

Instructions:

- Combine chia seeds, almond milk, and vanilla essence in a container. Refrigerate overnight.
- Before serving, top with a combination of berries. This pudding contains omega-3 fatty acids and antioxidants.

Cultivating a Positive Relationship with Food: Mindful Eating

Maintaining a pleasant connection with food is critical for both physical and emotional health. Mindful eating is a strong discipline that promotes an aware and deliberate attitude to eating. Individuals who are present and attentive at meals might build a healthy relationship with food and boost overall wellbeing.

Here are some important ideas and practices for mindful eating.

Mindful Awareness:

Begin by paying attention to your body's hunger and fullness signs. Eat when you're hungry, and quit when you're full.

Be aware of the flavors, textures, and scents of your meal. Engage all of your senses in the dining experience.

Slow down:

Take your time during mealtimes. Chew your meal deeply and enjoy every bite. This enables your body to indicate when it is full, reducing overeating.

Put down your utensils in between mouthful to help you pace yourself and become more conscious.

Remove distractions:

Turn off all electronic devices, including televisions and cellphones, during meals. Distractions can lead to thoughtless eating and a loss of awareness about what and how much you're eating.

Gratitude and appreciation:

Express your appreciation for the food on your plate and the labor that went into making it. This optimistic outlook might improve your whole dining experience.
Take a time to appreciate where your food comes from and the nutrients it contains.

Listen to your body.

Pay attention to your body's cues for hunger and fullness. Eat when you're physically hungry, and stop when you're full, even if there's still food on your plate.

Nonjudgmental Awareness:

Don't classify meals as "good" or "bad." Instead, consider how various meals make you feel and what nutritional advantages they provide.

Be kind to yourself if you indulge sometimes. Guilt and shame have a bad influence on your relationship with food.

Portion Control:

Pay attention to portion proportions and serve in moderate quantities. This helps to avoid overeating and allows you to eat a variety of meals in moderation.

Regular Check-Ins:

Check in with your hunger and fullness levels during mealtimes. This allows you to keep in tune with your body's signals and encourages a balanced eating style.

Practice gratitude:

Make a point of expressing thanks for your meals. Whether it's a simple acknowledgement or a minute of meditation, appreciating the nutrients you get may help you develop a healthy connection with food.

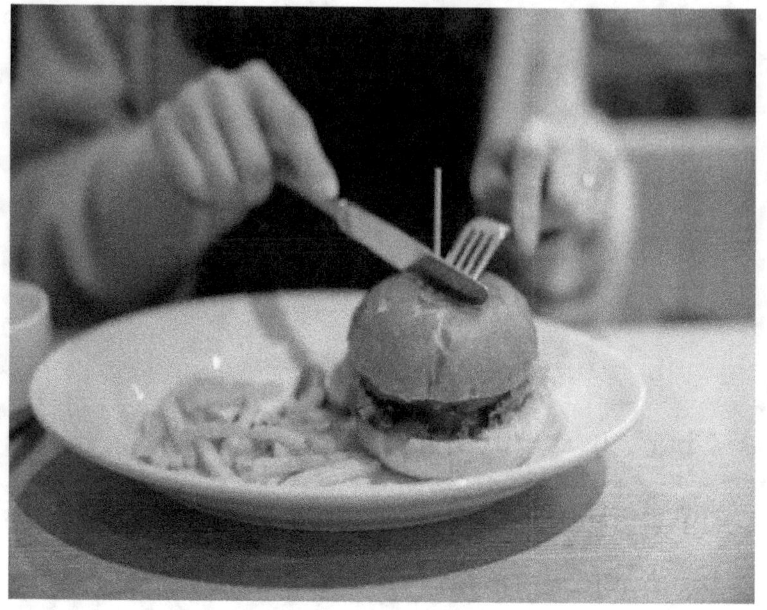

CHAPTER 4: SUPPORTING YOUR JOURNEY ON EVERY STEP

Addressing Common Fertility Challenges Through Food

Many people and couples throughout the world have fertility issues, which can cause mental and physical suffering. While medical therapies are essential for resolving fertility concerns, lifestyle variables, such as food, can have a substantial influence on reproductive health. Certain items in your diet may promote fertility and increase your chances of pregnancy. Here, we look at dietary options for typical reproductive issues.

Nutrient-Rich Foods:

Consuming a well-balanced diet rich in vital nutrients is critical to reproductive health. Key nutrients are:

Folate: Found in leafy greens, legumes, and fortified grains, folate is essential for fetal development and may increase fertility.

Omega-3 Fatty Acids: Cold-water fish, flaxseeds, and walnuts contain omega-3 fatty acids, which promote hormonal balance and may enhance egg quality.

Antioxidants: Berries, nuts, and vegetables are high in antioxidants, which assist to counteract oxidative stress, which can impair fertility.

Healthy fats:

Including sources of healthy fats in your diet is critical for hormone synthesis. Olive oil, avocados, and almonds are wonderful options for improving general reproductive health.

Lean proteins:

Choose lean protein sources such as poultry, fish, and plant-based alternatives such as lentils and quinoa. These proteins supply critical amino acids required for reproductive function.

Whole grains:

Instead of processed carbohydrates, choose for whole grains such as brown rice, oats, and quinoa. Whole grains provide complex carbs and fiber, which promote stable blood sugar levels and hormonal balance.

Limit processed foods and sugars:
Processed meals and excessive sugar consumption can cause inflammation and hormonal abnormalities. Choose natural, unprocessed foods to promote reproductive health.

Hydration:
Maintaining proper hydration is essential for general health, including reproductive

function. Water helps keep cervical mucous consistent, which aids sperm travel.

Moderate Caffeine and Alcohol Intake:

High caffeine and alcohol intake may have a detrimental influence on fertility. Moderate use is recommended, and some people may benefit from avoiding or limiting certain drugs.

Maintain a healthy weight:

Both being underweight and overweight might have an impact on fertility. Maintaining a healthy weight with a balanced diet and regular exercise can improve reproductive results.

Consideration of Specific Diets:

Some people may benefit from diets that are specifically customized to their requirements, such as the Mediterranean or fertility-focused diets. Consultation with a healthcare expert or nutritionist might give personalised advice.

Supplementation:

In some circumstances, supplements may be prescribed to correct particular nutritional deficits. However, it is critical to contact with a healthcare physician before beginning any supplements.

The Role of Supplements in Supporting Fertility

Fertility, or the capacity to conceive and carry a baby to term, is an essential component of reproductive health. While many variables influence fertility, including genetics, lifestyle, and general health, the function of supplements in fertility support has received more attention in recent years. In this article, we will look at the role of supplements in boosting reproductive health and their possible effect on fertility.

Nutrient deficiencies and fertility:
Nutrient shortages can have a substantial influence on fertility in both men and women. Vitamins and minerals are essential

for reproductive processes including ovulation, sperm production, and embryo development. Folic acid, vitamin D, zinc, and iron are some of the essential nutrients associated with fertility. Supplements can assist to correct these deficits and provide a more suitable environment for conception.

Antioxidants and Reproductive Health: Oxidative stress, generated by an imbalance of free radicals and antioxidants in the body, has been linked to infertility. Antioxidants such as vitamins C and E, selenium, and coenzyme Q10 assist to neutralize free radicals and protect reproductive cells from harm. Including antioxidant-rich supplements in one's diet may help to promote a healthy reproductive system.

Omega 3 Fatty Acids and Hormonal Balance:

Fish oil contains omega-3 fatty acids, mainly EPA and DHA, which are important for hormonal balance and inflammatory management. Hormonal abnormalities can interrupt a woman's menstrual cycle and a man's sperm production. Omega-3 supplements may help to boost hormone function, making the atmosphere more suitable to conception.

Herbal supplements and traditional medicines:

Some herbal supplements based on traditional medical methods have been linked to improved fertility. Vitex agnus-castus (chaste tree), maca root, and tribulus terrestris are all thought to improve hormonal balance and reproductive function. However, herbal supplements should be used with carefully and under the supervision of a healthcare practitioner.

Optimizing Male Fertility:

Male fertility is not only the responsibility of women; supplements can also help males optimize their reproductive health. Supplements such as zinc, selenium, vitamin

C, and coenzyme Q10 may improve the quality and quantity of sperm.

Consulting Healthcare Professionals:

Before introducing any supplements into a fertility-focused routine, talk with a healthcare provider. Individual health problems, medicines, and reproductive concerns differ, and a tailored approach ensures that supplements are both safe and effective.

Building a Team for Your Journey: Working with a Healthcare Professional.

Starting the path to enhance fertility is a big step, and putting together a supportive team is critical for success. A fertility specialist is a vital element of this team. This cooperation intends to use diet to increase fertility, establishing the groundwork for a healthier and more effective conception process.

Finding the Right Healthcare Professional: It is critical to select a healthcare provider who is knowledgeable about reproductive health and nutrition. Seek the advice of reproductive endocrinologists, fertility experts, or nutritionists who have expertise with fertility concerns. A thorough grasp of how diet affects reproductive health is required for developing individualized programs.

Schedule an initial appointment with a healthcare expert to discuss reproductive goals, medical history, and dietary habits. This encounter will provide a baseline and allow the professional to personalize their advice to your individual need.

Collaborate with a healthcare expert for a comprehensive nutritional examination. This might entail analyzing your current diet, detecting any dietary shortages, and evaluating lifestyle variables that may affect fertility. The objective is to have a good picture of your nutritional state and how it may affect fertility.

Work together to create a tailored nutrition plan based on the evaluation. This strategy should contain recommendations for certain nutrients known to promote fertility, such as folate, zinc, omega-3 fatty acids, and antioxidants. The healthcare expert will assist you in selecting dietary choices that are compatible with your reproductive goals.

Healthcare professionals have a crucial role in promoting education and empowerment as part of teamwork. Understanding how specific meals and minerals affect fertility allows you to make your own educated decisions. Regular check-ins and instructional sessions will boost your confidence in adhering to the prescribed nutritional plan.

Monitoring and Adjustments: Fertility and dietary requirements may alter over time. Regular monitoring, potentially via follow-up consultations and evaluations, enables the healthcare practitioner to make required changes to the dietary plan. This guarantees that the strategy remains in line with your changing requirements.

Healthcare professionals can recommend holistic lifestyle modifications that improve fertility, in addition to nutrition advice. Stress management tactics, exercise guidelines, and sleep hygiene may be used in addition to dietary treatments to provide a more holistic approach.

Maintain open conversation with your healthcare provider. A supportive and communicative connection will make the partnership more productive. Share your experiences, difficulties, and any changes in your health or lifestyle to obtain timely advice.

Conclusion

Finally, adopting a diet rich in authentic, nutritious foods has shown to be an effective tool for increasing fertility and general reproductive health. The complex interplay of nutrients contained in fresh fruits, vegetables, whole grains, lean proteins, and vital fats helps to maintain hormonal balance, improve reproductive function, and boost the likelihood of conception.

Individuals may equip their bodies with the building blocks for good reproductive health by selecting nutrient-dense alternatives and limiting their consumption of processed meals. The benefits of a true dietary approach go beyond fertility, improving general health and vigor.

Furthermore, eating a variety of colorful, plant-based meals provides a varied spectrum of vitamins, minerals, and antioxidants, all of which play important roles in reproductive processes. Equally crucial is the emphasis on keeping a healthy weight, as excess or inadequate body fat can disturb hormonal balance and impair fertility.

As we manage the difficulties of modern existence, we must recognize the need of real nourishment for fertility. This holistic approach not only tackles dietary concerns, but also promotes a lifestyle that promotes mental and emotional well-being, both of which are critical components of a successful reproductive journey.

Individuals who create a dedication to fueling their bodies with authentic, nutrient-rich meals not only increase their odds of conceiving, but also develop habits that encourage long-term health. Adopting a true food philosophy for fertility is a proactive and powerful step toward providing the best conditions for the miracle of life to occur.